C000149462

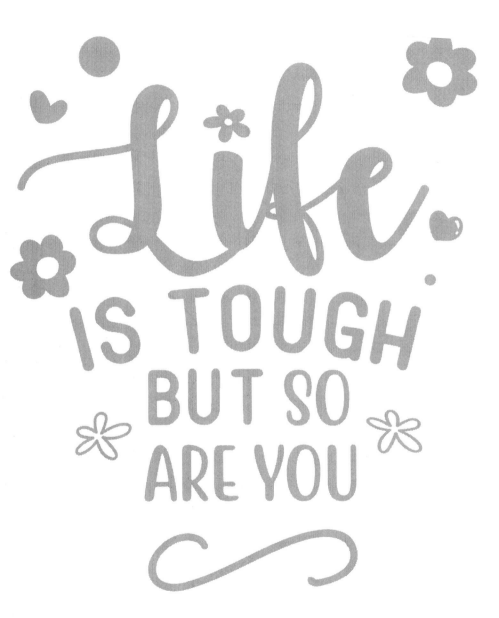

Copyright © 2022
All rights reserved
Seriously Simple Gratitude
brought to you by Rose Grace Press

THE IDEA BEHIND THIS JOURNAL

For years the idea of keeping a daily positivity journal seemed impossible. I wanted to feel grateful, but I could only think of all the negative things in my life.

With all that negativity in my mind, it's not surprising that I got sick. That's when I decided that I had to make some changes – one of which was to find a way to incorporate the habit of gratitude into my life.

I began looking for a way that would work for someone who, like myself, found it hard to find things to be grateful for.

That's when I came across the 'seriously simple gratitude" idea – and just like that, I found myself able to feel and express gratitude effortlessly.

And it can do the same for you. You'll be able to:

✓ make daily positivity an enjoyable habit, not a chore
✓ find dozens of things to be thankful for in moments
✓ start each day with positive thoughts

Inside you'll find everything you'll need to start your journey to positivity – and you'll discover this really works!

Are you ready to get started ?

SERIOUSLY SIMPLE GRATITUDE

When I came across this idea, I couldn't believe I hadn't heard of it before. It was so simple, yet so powerful. In a nutshell, this is how to harness the power of 'seriously simple gratitude'.

Imagine that you wake up tomorrow morning, with only the things you've been thankful for … what or who would you have around you?

Start by thinking about your bedroom. What would you miss if you woke up tomorrow morning and it wasn't there?

Here's a few of mine:

- ✓ warm duvet and pillows for a cozy sleep
- ✓ clothes I love in the wardrobe
- ✓ a radiator to keep me warm on cold nights

You get the idea! Each page has prompts to help you reflect and express your thanks for the things, experiences and people that you're grateful for. It's not rocket science, but it works.

Simply imagining that you woke up tomorrow morning without them can make you thankful for dozens of little things!

YOU ARE

Amazing,

remember

THAT

Thinking of my bedroom or the place where I sleep. What would I'd miss if it wasn't here?

_____

_____

_____

_____

_____

_____

_____

A favorite childhood memory:

To get you started: a trip to the beach, a vacation, Christmas?

_____

_____

_____

_____

_____

_____

_____

People I've enjoyed spending time with:

To get you started: friends, family, work colleagues ...

_____

_____

_____

_____

_____

_____

_____

Some positive aspects to where I live right now:

To get you started: is it close to shops, to nature or family?

_____

_____

_____

_____

_____

_____

_____

DAY: .... DATE ....

Foods I'm grateful for:

_____

_____

_____

_____

A food-related memory that makes me smile:

_____

_____

_____

Something I've enjoyed listening to or watching:

_____

_____

How can I take care of myself:

_____

_____

_____

_____

DAY: .... DATE ....

'm grateful for someone who encourages me:

_____

_____

_____

_____

Something I've appreciated seeing:

_____

_____

Someone that makes me smile:

_____

_____

_____

How can I take care of myself:

_____

_____

_____

_____

DAY: .... DATE ....

Today I'm grateful for these wonderful memories:

_____

_____

_____

_____

A vacation or trip I'm thankful to have experienced:

_____

_____

Small victories I had recently:

_____

_____

_____

How can I take care of myself today:

_____

_____

_____

_____

DAY: .... DATE ....

Today I'm grateful for my friends and family:

_____

_____

_____

_____

A friend I'm especially thankful for:

_____

_____

Something I noticed recently:

_____

_____

_____

How can I take care of myself:

_____

_____

_____

_____

DAY: .... DATE ....

I'm grateful for the simple things in life, including:

_____

_____

_____

_____

When I last saw a rainbow:

_____

_____

_____

Something that makes me feel cozy:

_____

_____

How can I take care of myself:

_____

_____

_____

_____

DAY: .... DATE ....

Today I'm grateful for my favorite foods:

_____

_____

_____

_____

I'm thankful for phone apps which make life easier:

_____

_____

Something someone gave me recently:

_____

_____

_____

How can I take care of myself today:

_____

_____

_____

_____

DAY: .... DATE ....

Today I'm grateful for music, especially:

_____

_____

_____

_____

Someone I'm thankful to have met:

_____

_____

I'm thankful for something I created:

_____

_____

_____

How can I take care of myself:

_____

_____

_____

_____

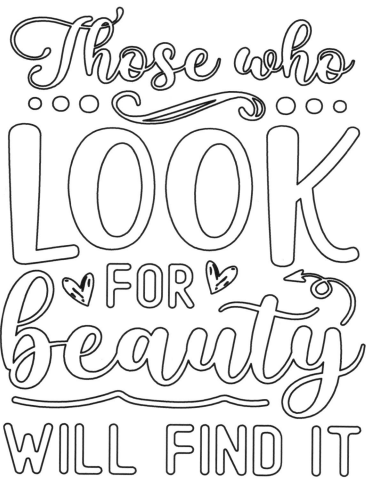

Some of my favorite foods:

To get you started: ice cream pizza,, chocolate, french fries …

_____

_____

_____

_____

_____

_____

A time when I made someone feel good:

To get you started: did you make someone laugh or smile …

_____

_____

_____

_____

_____

_____

List some people in your life that you are grateful for:

To get you started: a friend, a neighbor, a family member …

_____

_____

_____

_____

_____

_____

_____

List some people in your life who inspire you:

To get you started: a celebrity, an actor, a sports person …

_____

_____

_____

_____

_____

_____

DAY: .... DATE ....

Today I'm grateful for time spent with a friend:

_____

_____

_____

_____

A place I'm thankful to have visited:

_____

_____

Small victories I've had:

_____

_____

_____

How can I take care of myself today:

_____

_____

_____

_____

DAY: .... DATE ....

Today I'm grateful for friends and family, especially:

_____

_____

_____

_____

A friendship or relationship I'm thankful for:

_____

_____

Something I experienced recently:

_____

_____

_____

How can I take care of myself:

_____

_____

_____

DAY: .... DATE ....

TV shows I'm thankful for:

_____

_____

_____

_____

Something I enjoyed listening to:

_____

_____

A travel-related memory that makes me smile:

_____

_____

_____

How can I take care of myself:

_____

_____

_____

_____

DAY: .... DATE ....

I'm grateful for someone who appreciates me:

_____

_____

_____

_____

Something I appreciated seeing recently:

_____

_____

Someone who makes me smile:

_____

_____

_____

How can I take care of myself:

_____

_____

_____

_____

DAY: .... DATE ....

Today I'm grateful for music, including:

_____

_____

_____

_____

Somewhere I'm thankful to have visited:

_____

_____

I'm thankful for something I've experienced:

_____

_____

_____

How can I take care of myself:

_____

_____

_____

_____

DAY: .... DATE ....

I'm grateful for the simple things in life, such as:

_____

_____

_____

_____

Someone who makes me feel special:

_____

_____

When did you last see the moon and the stars?

_____

_____

_____

How can I take care of myself:

_____

_____

_____

_____

DAY: .... DATE ....

Today I'm grateful for TV shows or movies:

_____

_____

_____

_____

I'm thankful for technology which make life easier:

_____

_____

Something someone said to me recently:

_____

_____

_____

How can I take care of myself today:

_____

_____

_____

_____

Sometimes COURAGE

MEANS HOLDING ON

Sometimes COURAGE

MEANS LETTING GO

Someone who has helped me grow or learn new things

To get you started: a teacher, a grandparent, aunt or uncle …

_____

_____

_____

_____

_____

_____

_____

The kindest thing anyone has done for me:

To get you started: a gift, a thoughtful deed, time spent …

_____

_____

_____

_____

_____

_____

_____

What achievements am I proud of?

To get you started: an academic achievement, a challenge you overcame …

_____

_____

_____

_____

_____

_____

_____

What have people said to me or about me that made me feel good?

_____

_____

_____

_____

_____

_____

_____

DAY: .... DATE ....

I'm thankful for these things I couldn't live without:

_____

_____

_____

_____

Something I enjoyed watching:

_____

_____

A family memory that makes me smile:

_____

_____

_____

How can I take care of myself:

_____

_____

_____

_____

DAY: .... DATE ....

I'm grateful for someone who accepts me as I am:

_____

_____

_____

_____

Something I was able to do:

_____

_____

Something that makes me happy:

_____

_____

_____

How can I take care of myself:

_____

_____

_____

_____

DAY: .... DATE ....

Today I'm grateful for people that love me, especially:

_____

_____

_____

_____

Someone I'm thankful to have in my life:

_____

_____

I'm thankful for someone who messaged or called:

_____

_____

_____

How can I take care of myself:

_____

_____

_____

_____

AY: .... DATE ....

'm grateful for the simple things in life, such as:

_____

_____

_____

_____

Someone that makes me feel appreciated:

_____

_____

A time when I enjoyed the warm sun on my skin?

_____

_____

_____

How can I take care of myself:

_____

_____

_____

_____

DAY: .... DATE ....

I'm grateful for technology that helps me keep in touch with family and friends, especially:

_____

_____

_____

_____

I'm thankful for household technology that makes life easier, including:

_____

_____

Something someone said to me recently:

_____

_____

_____

How can I take care of myself:

_____

_____

_____

DAY: .... DATE ....

Today I'm grateful for fond memories of this person:

_____

_____

_____

_____

A show, movie or concert I'm thankful to have seen:

_____

_____

Small victories I've had recently:

_____

_____

_____

How can I take care of myself:

_____

_____

_____

_____

DAY: .... DATE ....

I'm grateful for friends and family, especially:

_____

_____

_____

_____

I'm especially thankful for the ability to be able to:

_____

_____

Something I enjoyed recently:

_____

_____

_____

How can I take care of myself today:

_____

_____

_____

Don't give up on yourself

Thinking of a mistake I once made. How has it helped me to become a better person?

_____

_____

_____

_____

_____

_____

_____

Something I really hoped was going to happen. It didn't, but it worked out for the best:

_____

_____

_____

_____

_____

_____

_____

Some modern comforts I'm thankful for:

To get you started: running water, electricity …

_____

_____

_____

_____

_____

_____

_____

Animals or pets I love or appreciate:

To get you started: a pet, horses, whales, lions, giraffes …

_____

_____

_____

_____

_____

_____

DAY: .... DATE ....

TV shows or movies I've enjoyed recently:

_____

_____

_____

_____

Phone apps I use to keep in touch:

_____

_____

Something helpful I learned recently:

_____

_____

_____

How can I take care of myself:

_____

_____

_____

DAY: .... DATE ....

Vacation memories I'm thankful for:

_____

_____

_____

_____

One of my favorite vacation memories:

_____

_____

Small victories I've had this week:

_____

_____

_____

How can I take care of myself:

_____

_____

_____

_____

DAY: .... DATE ....

Friends and family I'm grateful for today:

_____

_____

_____

_____

Someone I'm especially thankful for:

_____

_____

Someone or something I said no to recently:

_____

_____

_____

How can I take care of myself:

_____

_____

_____

_____

DAY: .... DATE ....

Foods I enjoyed recently:

_____

_____

_____

_____

Something I've enjoyed doing:

_____

_____

A childhood memory that makes me smile:

_____

_____

_____

How can I take care of myself:

_____

_____

_____

_____

DAY: .... DATE ....

Someone I'm thankful for today:

_____

_____

_____

Something I appreciated being able to do :

_____

_____

Something that I find comforting:

_____

_____

_____

How can I take care of myself:

_____

_____

_____

_____

DAY: .... DATE ....

Today I'm grateful for music that I love, especially:

_____

_____

_____

_____

Someone I'm thankful to have met:

_____

_____

Something I'm thankful for which doesn't cost money:

_____

_____

_____

How can I take care of myself:

_____

_____

_____

_____

DAY: .... DATE ....

I'm grateful for the simple things in life, such as:

_____

_____

_____

_____

When did you last enjoy a coffee, tea or hot chocolate?

_____

_____

What changes have you made that you're thankful for?

_____

_____

_____

How can I take care of myself today:

_____

_____

_____

_____

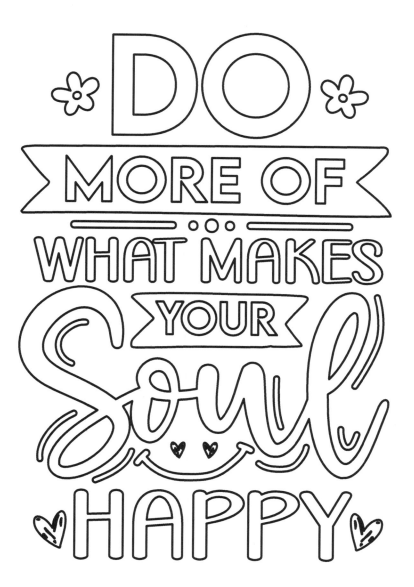

DO
MORE OF
WHAT MAKES
YOUR
Soul
HAPPY

What things do I do that make me lose track of time?

To get you started: making, baking or creating something ...

_____

_____

_____

_____

_____

_____

What have I enjoyed making, doing or creating?

To get you started: coloring, knitting, planning a vacation ...

_____

_____

_____

_____

_____

_____

What things make my soul happy?

To get you started: being in nature, being with family ...

_____

_____

_____

_____

_____

_____

_____

How might I do more of what makes my soul happy in the next few days or weeks?

_____

_____

_____

_____

_____

_____

_____

DAY: .... DATE ....

I loved watching these TV shows or movies as a child:

_____

_____

_____

_____

I'm thankful for a small gesture:

_____

_____

What well-known person are you grateful for?

_____

_____

_____

How can I take care of myself:

_____

_____

_____

_____

DAY: .... DATE ....

What was the best gift you've ever received and why?

_____

_____

_____

_____

The season I most look forward to each year:

_____

_____

Small victories I've had:

_____

_____

_____

How can I take care of myself:

_____

_____

_____

_____

DAY: .... DATE ....

Today I'm grateful for the positive people in my life:

_____

_____

_____

_____

Someone I'm especially thankful for:

_____

_____

Someone that's helped me:

_____

_____

_____

How can I take care of myself:

_____

_____

_____

_____

DAY: .... DATE ....

The abilities I'm grateful for:

_____

_____

_____

_____

The thing I most enjoy about nature:

_____

_____

A scientific discovery I'm thankful for:

_____

_____

_____

How can I take care of myself:

_____

_____

_____

_____

DAY: .... DATE ....

This is a quote that encourages me:

_____

_____

_____

_____

Somewhere I feel most relaxed:

_____

_____

A podcast or video that I've enjoyed:

_____

_____

_____

How can I take care of myself:

_____

_____

_____

_____

DAY: .... DATE ....

Today I'm grateful for people I love, especially:

_____

_____

_____

_____

A little luxury I'm thankful for:

_____

_____

I'm thankful that I learned:

_____

_____

_____

How can I take care of myself:

_____

_____

_____

_____

DAY: .... DATE ....

I'm grateful for everyday objects, including:

_____

_____

_____

A time in my life when I felt really happy:

_____

_____

Something in my home that brings me joy:

_____

_____

_____

How can I take care of myself today:

_____

_____

_____

great things
—NEVER— come
from your
COMFORT ZONE

When have I seen others out of their comfort zone, where it turned out positively?

_____

_____

_____

_____

_____

_____

What things have I done that were out of my comfort zone, that turned out better than expected?

_____

_____

_____

_____

_____

_____

What small success am I proud of today?

To get you started: getting out of bed, taking a walk …

_____

_____

_____

_____

_____

_____

_____

Which people or beliefs inspire me to keep going?

To get you started: someone famous, a friend or loved one …

_____

_____

_____

_____

_____

_____

_____

DAY: .... DATE ....

One good thing that happened to me:

_____

_____

_____

Something I accomplished recently:

_____

_____

An opportunity that I'm grateful to have had:

_____

_____

_____

How can I take care of myself:

_____

_____

_____

_____

DAY: .... DATE ....

The three items I'd take with me to a desert island:

_____

_____

_____

_____

A guilty pleasure I'm grateful for:

_____

_____

Small victories I've had:

_____

_____

_____

How can I take care of myself:

_____

_____

_____

_____

DAY: .... DATE ....

Something I love about a friend or family member:

_____

_____

_____

My favorite part of the day is usually:

_____

_____

Something I saw today:

_____

_____

_____

How can I take care of myself:

_____

_____

_____

DAY: .... DATE ....

Music I'm thankful for:

_____

_____

_____

_____

Something I enjoyed eating recently:

_____

_____

A freedom I'm thankful to have:

_____

_____

_____

How can I take care of myself:

_____

_____

_____

_____

DAY: .... DATE ....

I'm grateful for someone who's helped me in the past:

_____

_____

_____

_____

Something I appreciated seeing:

_____

_____

Someone that makes me smile:

_____

_____

_____

How can I take care of myself:

_____

_____

_____

_____

DAY: .... DATE ....

I'm grateful for the obsession my country has about:

_____

_____

_____

_____

Somewhere in my country I'm thankful to have seen:

_____

_____

Some positive news I heard recently:

_____

_____

_____

How can I take care of myself:

_____

_____

_____

_____

DAY: .... DATE ....

When did you play your favorite music track? What is it called and who is it by?

.:
_____

_____

_____

_____

A meaningful gift I've received:

_____

_____

I'm grateful for the sacrifices this person made for me:

_____

_____

_____

How can I take care of myself today:

_____

_____

_____

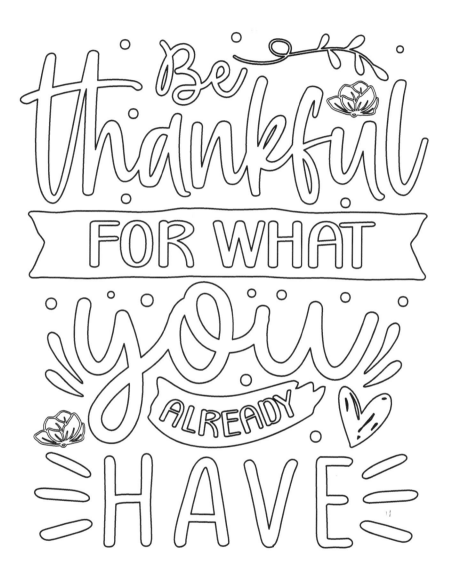

Some items of technology I'm thankful for:

To get you started: TV, mobile phone, cars ...

_____

_____

_____

_____

_____

_____

Some books, TV or movies I've enjoyed:

To get you started: a movie you've watched over and over ...

_____

_____

_____

_____

_____

_____

_____

Someone who's been with me or supported me during some of my most difficult times?

_____

_____

_____

_____

_____

_____

_____

Something money can't buy that I'm grateful for:

To get you started: friendship, respect, trust …

_____

_____

_____

_____

_____

_____

_____

DAY: .... DATE ....

I'm grateful that these small things make me happy:

_____

_____

_____

I'm thankful for a song that makes me feel happy:

_____

_____

I'm thankful for a good deed I've seen or experienced:

_____

_____

_____

How can I take care of myself:

_____

_____

_____

DAY: .... DATE ....

Today I'm grateful for these childhood memories:

_____

_____

_____

_____

One of the best meals I've ever cooked:

_____

_____

One of the best meals I've ever eaten:

_____

_____

_____

How can I take care of myself:

_____

_____

_____

_____

DAY: .... DATE ....

A time in my life when I did something scary and it turned out OK:

_____

_____

_____

_____

A luxury I'm thankful for:

_____

_____

Something I'm thankful to have today that I didn't have a year ago:

_____

_____

_____

How can I take care of myself:

_____

_____

_____

_____

DAY: .... DATE ....

Writers, musicians or artists I'm thankful for:

_____
_____
_____
_____

Something I enjoyed seeing:

_____
_____

Thinking of a photo that I love, who or what does it make me feel grateful for?

_____
_____
_____

How can I take care of myself:

_____
_____
_____
_____

DAY: .... DATE ....

A teacher, colleague or mentor I'm grateful for :

_____

_____

_____

Something I appreciated seeing :

_____

_____

A personality trait I'm proud of:

_____

_____

_____

How can I take care of myself:

_____

_____

_____

DAY: .... DATE ....

When I've had a rough day, what cheers me up is:

_____

_____

_____

_____

Somewhere amazing I visited that I will never forget:

_____

_____

What I most enjoy about this season:

_____

_____

_____

How can I take care of myself:

_____

_____

_____

_____

DAY: .... DATE ....

I'm grateful for hobbies I've enjoyed, including:

_____

_____

_____

_____

People that know me say that I'm good at this:

_____

_____

My favorite spot in my neighborhood:

_____

_____

_____

How can I take care of myself today:

_____

_____

_____

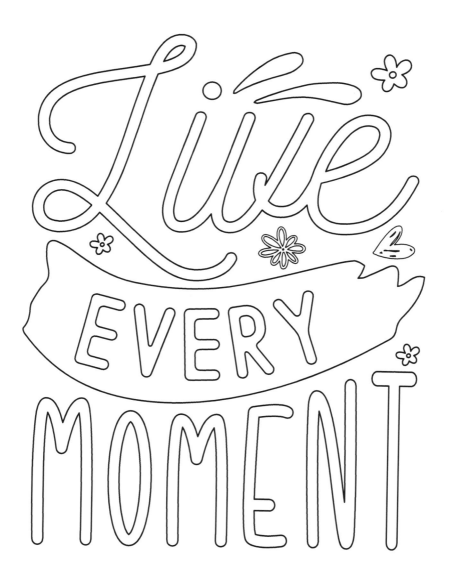

What signs of the seasons have I seen lately?

To get you started: leaves, flowers, trees, weather …

_____

_____

_____

_____

_____

_____

_____

When did I last spend time out in nature?
How did it make me feel?

_____

_____

_____

_____

_____

_____

_____

Things I noticed when I went outside recently:

To get you started: people, change of season, bright lights …

_____

_____

_____

_____

_____

_____

_____

What types of weather do you most enjoy?

To get you started: sunshine, thunderstorms …

_____

_____

_____

_____

_____

_____

_____

DAY: .... DATE ....

I'm grateful for this aspect of my upbringing:

_____

_____

_____

_____

I'm thankful for someone who was kind to me recently:

_____

_____

The most beautiful place I've ever been to:

_____

_____

_____

How can I take care of myself:

_____

_____

_____

_____

DAY: .... DATE ....

The highlight of my week this week:

_____

_____

_____

_____

A quality I admire in a friend or family member:

_____

_____

Small victories I've had:

_____

_____

_____

How can I take care of myself:

_____

_____

_____

_____

DAY: .... DATE ....

Things I love about where I live:

_____

_____

_____

_____

Something I own that makes life easier:

_____

_____

Something I enjoyed recently:

_____

_____

_____

How can I take care of myself:

_____

_____

_____

_____

DAY: .... DATE ....

Things about the world around me I'm grateful for:

_____

_____

_____

_____

Of my five senses, I'm most grateful for:

_____

_____

An article of clothing I'll never part with:

_____

_____

_____

How can I take care of myself:

_____

_____

_____

_____

DAY: .... DATE ....

My favorite desserts include:

_____

_____

_____

Something I enjoyed eating recently:

_____

_____

A quote or Bible verse that has special meaning to me:

_____

_____

_____

How can I take care of myself:

_____

_____

_____

DAY: .... DATE ....

My favorite memory from last year:

_____

_____

_____

_____

An invention I'm thankful for:

_____

_____

I'm thankful for my favorite colors, especially:

_____

_____

_____

How can I take care of myself:

_____

_____

_____

_____

DAY: .... DATE ....

The life experience that's had the biggest positive impact on me:

_____

_____

_____

_____

Someone who cares about how I'm feeling:

_____

_____

Stress-relieving items I'm thankful for:

_____

_____

_____

How can I take care of myself today:

_____

_____

_____

_____

KINDNESS IS FREE

Something kind or thoughtful that's happened to me recently:

_____

_____

_____

_____

_____

_____

What kindness or thoughtfulness have I been able to show others recently?

_____

_____

_____

_____

_____

_____

Five people that make me feel happy or loved:

**Someone I know that is always appreciative
or grateful. What do I most appreciate about them?**

DAY: .... DATE ....

I'm grateful for animals and pets, especially:

_____

_____

_____

I'm thankful that I got to walk or hike here:

_____

_____

A store I like shopping in:

_____

_____

_____

How can I take care of myself:

_____

_____

_____

DAY: .... DATE ....

I'm grateful for a fun trip I took:

_____

_____

_____

_____

A time I was able to pamper myself:

_____

_____

Small victories I had lately:

_____

_____

_____

How can I take care of myself:

_____

_____

_____

_____

DAY: .... DATE ....

I'm thankful for people who've helped me:

_____

_____

_____

A friendship I'm especially thankful for:

_____

_____

The best thing I ever bought:

_____

_____

_____

How can I take care of myself:

_____

_____

_____

_____

DAY: .... DATE ....

Ways technology has helped me this week:

_____

_____

_____

_____

Something that brightened my day recently:

_____

_____

A smell that brings back fond memories:

_____

_____

_____

How can I take care of myself:

_____

_____

_____

_____

DAY: .... DATE ....

I'm grateful for someone who believes in me:

_____

_____

_____

_____

A role model who inspires me:

_____

_____

My favorite ice cream flavors:

_____

_____

_____

How can I take care of myself:

_____

_____

_____

_____

DAY: .... DATE ....

Some skills I'm thankful to have:

_____

_____

_____

_____

A positive experience I'm thankful for:

_____

_____

Material comforts I'm thankful for today:

_____

_____

_____

How can I take care of myself:

_____

_____

_____

_____

DAY: .... DATE ....

Someone I'm grateful for today:

_____

_____

_____

Something that I love about my home:

_____

_____

Something small that makes my life better:

_____

_____

_____

How can I take care of myself today:

_____

_____

_____

AT THE END OF THE DAY
ALL you need
· IS HOPE ·
&
Strength,
HOPE THAT IT WILL
Get better
And
Strength
TO HOLD ON UNTIL IT DOES

Self Care Suggestions

Here's some ideas to get you started:

- ✓ listen to music
- ✓ enjoy a relaxing bath or refreshing shower
- ✓ get creative
- ✓ watch or listen to something that makes you laugh
- ✓ spend time with loved ones
- ✓ Enjoy a hot chocolate or coffee
- ✓ spend time alone
- ✓ meditate
- ✓ set boundaries
- ✓ spend time with supportive people
- ✓ take a walk
- ✓ spend time in nature
- ✓ say no to things which will add stress to your life
- ✓ unplug from social media
- ✓ treat yourself to a brownie
- ✓ be kind to yourself

There's some space on the next few pages for some suggestions of your own.

Why not make a note of some now, so you have them ready for the days when you might need a few ideas?

"Small"
Steps
ARE ALSO
Progress

strength GROWS IN THE moments WHEN YOU THINK you can't go on, BUT YOU KEEP going

Printed in Great Britain
by Amazon

28716847R00059